Dialysis *YOUR* Way

How to actively participate in your dialysis
treatment to maintain your well-being

By Antonio Richardson

Editing and Design by Susana M. Choy
Illustrations by Christina Rubalcava

ISBN-13: 978-1546970699
ISBN-10: 154697069X

Printed in the United States of America

Cover & Interior design © 2017 by Susana M. Choy
Illustrations © 2017 by Christina Rubalcava

First Edition

This book is dedicated to Ramona Wong.

Thank you for saving my life
and being my best friend.

Forward

Antonio has written a wonderful book describing his reluctant journey on dialysis. He describes how he took control of the process rather than letting it take control of him. Dialysis is a mechanical process, yet it involves human interaction with the machine. The technicians connect the patient to the machine, and the patient interacts with the technician and the machine. How the patient responds to both determines in part the final outcome. Read this delightful book, and it will give you the confidence to determine your own fate.

Roland Ng, MD, FACP

Table of Contents

Introduction

Hi everybody, my name is Antonio Richardson. The purpose of writing this book is to provide you with important information I learned while on hemodialysis from June 2004 to June 2011. My hemodialysis was performed in a dialysis center three times a week. I have no formal medical training. In fact, I was one of those people who hardly went to the doctor prior to receiving an abnormal laboratory report.

In this book, I will take you on a journey based on my experiences. I will address some of the challenges and complications that I experienced while prolonging my life on hemodialysis and share lessons learned from those experiences.

It is my hope that this information will help those who are currently on dialysis as well as those who have been diagnosed with Chronic Kidney Disease (CKD) and those who are not yet on dialysis.

The journey can get difficult at times and it certainly helps to have some insight about what's going on with your body from a veteran of dialysis who has already traveled down that road and survived.

This is from me to all of you, especially those with CKD.

Best wishes,

Antonio Richardson

Chapter 1

The Hemodialysis Bloodstream Catheter

The hemodialysis bloodstream catheter is for emergency use only! I want to be very clear about my opening statement about the catheter. The definition of an emergency in my case, was the need to initiate hemodialysis within the first week of meeting my kidney specialist, also called a nephrologist. Because my primary care doctor referred me to the nephrologist too late to proactively prepare for dialysis, a hemodialysis bloodstream catheter was the only option available to save my life.

This catheter is a plastic tube that the doctor put through my skin and into one of the large, major veins in my neck area to allow dirty blood to be filtered outside my body, which is what hemodialysis does. That meant one end of this plastic tube sat in my bloodstream, while the other end of the tube hung out of my neck, for six months.

From what I've learned, the need for immediate dialysis can come suddenly, especially if you already have reduced kidney function (CKD). If there has been no proactive preparation in creating a working fistula before the need for dialysis, then the situation would be a qualified emergency indication for a bloodstream catheter.

The catheter will save your life in that it allows for immediate dialysis. However, it comes with a lot of potentially serious problems. Here is a list of some of the problems I experienced with the hemodialysis catheter:

1. INFECTION. It was not a question of IF my hemodialysis catheter would get infected but a question of WHEN.

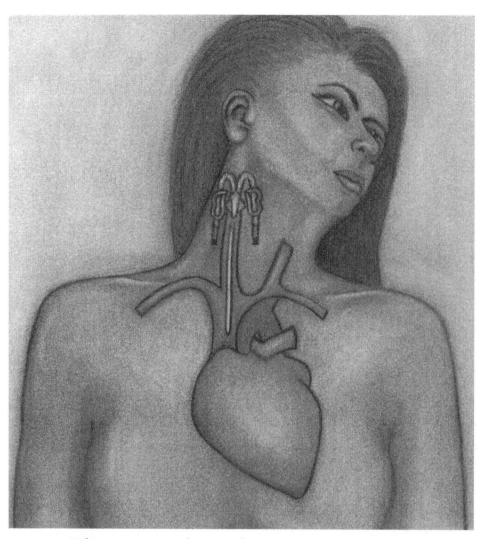

When using a catheter, it's not a question of IF my hemodialysis catheter would get infected but a question of WHEN.

My dialysis catheter got infected after only one month of use. I learned from my doctor that I didn't do anything to cause it. Simply having a dialysis catheter connected to my bloodstream automatically put me at risk for getting an infection of the catheter as well as a blood infection. I had no idea at the time that this meant my entire bloodstream could be infected with bacteria, which turned out to be the case. It could have killed me. The name of the bacteria that caused my infection was the mighty MRSA, or Methicillin Resistant Staphylococcus Aureus.

MRSA is a strain of bacteria that requires antibiotics stronger than the first line of antibiotics because it is resistant to the first line of antibiotics. Infections can occur more easily, frequently and can be more severe in people with weakened immune systems such as people on dialysis. MRSA can be found hanging around hospitals, nursing homes as well as dialysis centers. In fact, MRSA can be found anywhere, and once it entered my body through my hemodialysis catheter, it was scary.

My bloodstream infection resulted from using a hemodialysis catheter because the catheter provided bacteria an entryway straight into my bloodstream. A bloodstream infection is a very serious medical condition.

Remembering my catheter bloodstream infection, I first felt the symptoms while actually on hemodialysis. First, I felt chills. Then, when my body started to shake uncontrollably, I reported it to a nurse. She put a thermometer in my mouth and found I had a fever. She contacted my nephrologist, took blood samples for a blood culture and gave me an antibiotic through my blood line. The samples that came back a few days later revealed I had a MRSA infection. I was admitted into the hospital immediately following the completion of my dialysis session. At first, the fever wouldn't go away, so they removed the infected catheter and replaced it with a new one before my next dialysis was needed, while continuing to give me antibiotics. My fever finally went down the next day.

I could have been hospitalized for days even weeks depending on how things progressed. Fortunately, I was still young and pretty fit so I didn't have to stay in the hospital for more than a few days.

Be aware that while hospitalized, you will be surrounded by a lot of other people with infections who are being treated with antibiotics. Because you have a weakened immune system as a dialysis patient, you are at increased risk for catching other infections that may worsen your condition. Infections can kill and that's another reason why I try hard to stay out of hospitals.

I learned that regular exercise and good nutrition helps my body remain strong which also decreases my likelihood of being admitted into the hospital. But when I needed to be hospitalized, I knew the extra strength also helped me respond to treatment quicker, heal faster and get discharged sooner.

After being discharged from the hospital for my MRSA catheter and bloodstream infection, my nephrologist ordered the dialysis nurses to continue the course of antibiotics for six weeks. I had no issues during those six weeks but during the very next dialysis treatment after finishing the antibiotics, I felt a chill and started shaking, just like the first time. The nurse said I had a fever again, called my nephrologist, got blood cultures, and I ended up being prescribed the same course of antibiotics for another six weeks. It was MRSA that grew in that second batch of blood cultures too.

This happened all over again when they tried to stop the antibiotic a second time after what was now a total of twelve weeks of antibiotic treatment! My doctor said the bacteria was probably holding onto the catheter in my bloodstream. It wasn't until they could use my fistula — a more viable alternative to the neck catheter — six months later that the MRSA was finally killed off and I began to really feel well while on dialysis.

2. LACK OF GOOD BLOOD CLEANING. My catheter was

doing the most important job of allowing me to have the hemodialysis treatments and thereby saving my life. However, my catheter would not allow the dialysis machine to clean my blood adequately. What I mean by this is that my dialysis sessions were not meeting the standard level of blood cleaning. The dialysis center's standard was to clean all dialysis patients' blood at a minimum of 70%. It was reported for months that my blood was cleaned only 60 – 67%. The day after dialysis I would still sometimes feel nauseated, drowsy and tired. I was told that because the catheter had a limit to how fast the blood flowed through the system, the only way to get better cleaning while using a catheter was to increase the length of my treatment or to upgrade to a larger dialyzer (the blood filter). The upgrade to a larger dialyzer did not happen for a couple of months due to the dialysis center's body weight criteria. Since I didn't weigh enough, my request for a larger dialyzer was not immediately granted.

My nephrologist increased my time on dialysis from four hours to four hours and forty five minutes. This helped. My nephrologist always said that the longer you dialyze, the more gentle and complete a dialysis treatment you will have, and the longer you might live.

It was about two months later when I finally got my larger dialyzer. Things did get better for me in that I no longer felt the nausea, drowsiness and fatigue the day after dialysis. However, I didn't feel much better until I got rid of the hemodialysis catheter and started using my fistula. My blood flowed faster using the larger passageway my fistula provided and this allowed better cleaning for the remaining years that I was on hemodialysis.

I was on hemodialysis for a total of seven years.

3. CATHETER CARE. One of the first things I did after getting my hemodialysis catheter and having the surgery for my fistula, was to eliminate all contact sports from my life because a simple fall or accidentally banging my arm against any solid object could possibly damage my fistula. Another concern was keeping my catheter dry because in the event it got wet, an infection was almost sure to follow. This meant that instead of taking a shower, I needed to bathe from the bathroom sink with a washcloth.

A dialysis nurse would clean my catheter each time I went to dialysis. They will do the same for you should you have a catheter. The cleaning solution they used was Betadine.

Be advised. ... You may unknowingly carry a Betadine odor with you around the clock. Since I wasn't allowed to wet or wash that area, and Betadine was reapplied during every hemodialysis session, I sure did. It was months after my catheter was removed that a close friend told me I carried a Betadine odor with me the whole time the hemodialysis catheter was there. I used to wonder why nobody wanted to sit next to me on the bus when there was an open seat.

The dialysis catheter is normally placed into the jugular vein on either side of the neck. Depending on which version of the catheter you receive, it may be seen from the outside of your shirt.

If you are employed and your employment duties require physical labor, you may be determined to be a liability and possibly laid off as a result.

Here's something to keep in mind. ... You're going to have to make many adjustments in your new life on dialysis. It is very important that things get off to a good, smooth start. So when your nephrologist recommends you get a fistula, DON'T WAIT. To avoid what I went through, schedule an appointment with the surgeon based on availability but I would strongly suggest that this gets done within 30 days of your nephrologist's recommendation.

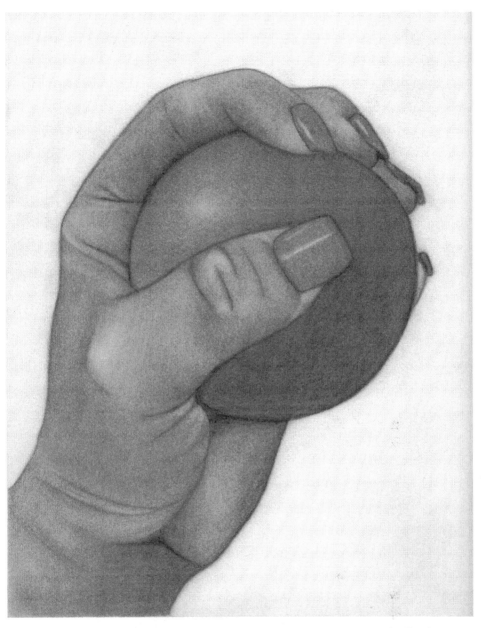

I was given a squeeze ball, about the size of a tennis ball, that I would squeeze in sets of 10. Exercises like this is one of the usual ways to help a fistula mature.

Chapter 2

The Fistula

The fistula is a surgically created connection between an artery and vein. It is the access way most nephrologists want their patients to have for hemodialysis. The fistula requires less maintenance than the hemodialysis catheter, carries less risk for infection and can be very reliable.

Having a good vein is a must for a fistula and creating a good, reliable fistula requires some work on the patient's behalf.

I recall when I got my fistula. ... I wasn't allowed to use it right away because it had to be developed through exercise. The vascular surgeon who performed the procedure called the shots as to when it could be used. In spite of my almost continuous catheter infection, the surgeon prevented the dialysis technician from using my fistula for six months. This was after repeated calls to the vascular surgeon by my nephrologist to report my recurring catheter bloodstream infections and to request permission to use it. The surgeon felt the fistula was too immature to be used for the first six months, meaning it was not big enough and the walls of the vein had not strengthened enough. If needles are put into a fistula before it is mature, it could cause it to leak or to collapse.

To strengthen and help the fistula mature, I was given a squeeze ball, about the size of a tennis ball, that I would squeeze in sets of 10. Exercising like this helped my fistula vein mature faster. I made sure I squeezed the ball at least 100 times prior to going to bed every night.

Since I want my fistula to be my lifetime life line, allowing access to my bloodstream for hemodialysis, my nephrologist advised me not to get repeated needle pokes around the same area, which could weaken the vein wall. I needed to protect the fistula vein wall from possibly

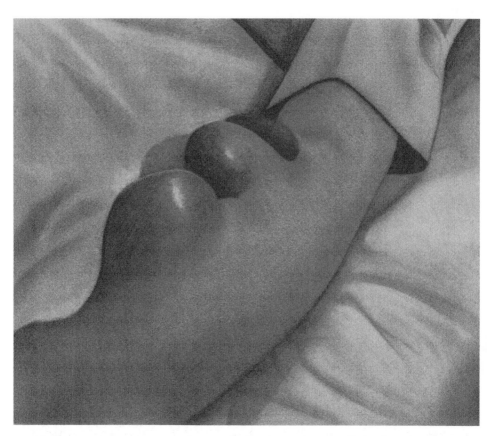

Have you ever seen a person who is on hemodialysis who has one or more lumps on their fistula arm about the size of a golf ball? Those are aneurysms and could be a direct result of the dialysis technicians placing needles into the same area of the fistula repeatedly.

being abused, because weakening the wall could cause thinning, stretching and eventually an aneurysm of the fistula.

Before each dialysis session my arm would still be puffy and sore from the needle stick performed during my previous dialysis session. Keep in mind that the dialysis technicians rotated each week in my dialysis center so I often did not see the same technician who put me on the machine again for weeks, sometimes over a month. Because of the rotation schedule, I realized they didn't know my body and it was up to me to SPEAK UP! Therefore, I would tell the dialysis technician that the area of the last needle stick was still sore and then show them where I wanted them to stick the needle for that session. I would walk them all the way up my vein for needle placement before returning back to the lowest site, and walk them up again.

After seven years on dialysis there is an area of six inches on my arm that shows a scar but no aneurysms from the dialysis needle sticks. Still, it's noticeable and sometimes people will ask me what caused it. I have to admit that I am very pleased with the way it looks after seven years of use.

By managing the needle placement with the dialysis technician I never got an aneurysm. Have you ever seen a person who is on hemodialysis who has one or more lumps on their fistula arm about the size of a golf ball? This could be a direct result of the dialysis technicians placing needles into the same swollen area of the fistula repeatedly. The reason why the technician might do this is that they are almost guaranteed to hit the vein they are looking for.

I spoke up to let the dialysis technicians know that I will always show them where to stick my needles. On a typical day at dialysis, prior to being put on the machine, the technician would say, "Hello, Mr. Richardson. Where do you want your needles stuck and how much water do you want taken off?"

The dialysis staff appreciated that I was taking an active role in my dialysis treatment. They were grateful that I was trying to assist in order to ensure that my dialysis treatments were successful and that I felt as well as I should at the end of each dialysis treatment session.

One final and important note about the fistula is the timing of when to get the surgery to create one. I've learned that there is a medical practice guideline that recommends that only when your GFR (Glomerular Filtration Rate) drops to 20, is it time to create a fistula. GFR is a calculation based on a blood test that roughly estimates the percentage of kidney function you have left.

The lead time between creating the fistula and starting dialysis is very important. After my fistula was created, I had six months of work squeezing the ball to help the fistula mature enough before my vascular surgeon would give the okay for use. Some people have told me that it took them a whole year or more for their fistula to mature. So it helps if you get this done and prepared for use ahead of time. Having a fistula will make starting hemodialysis easier and it doesn't carry the risks and problems of a hemodialysis bloodstream catheter.

Do your best to remember that once your GFR drops to 20 or below, traumatic things that happen to the body can cause the GFR to quickly fall further, possibly into end-stage kidney failure. Events like having a bad case of the flu, developing pneumonia, having a heart attack, or developing a tooth infection; yes, a tooth infection, could make your GFR drop.

So when your GFR is 20 or below, if your nephrologist is not scheduling for you to get a fistula, ask him/her if it makes sense to do so. This is another time you can speak up if you're willing to consider hemodialysis should your kidneys fail.

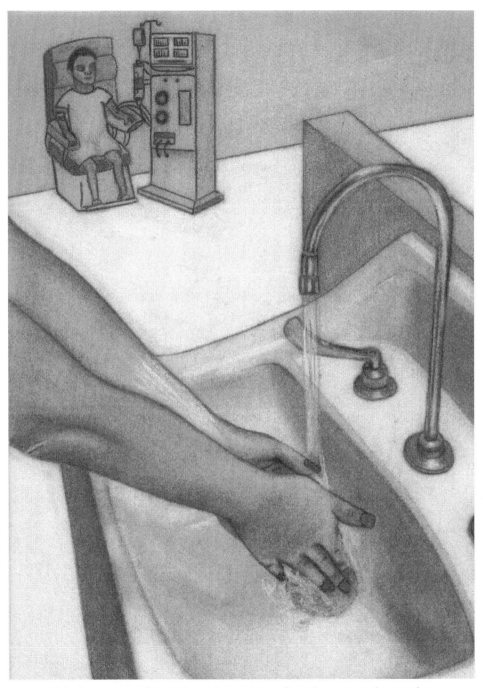

I would always wash my hands and my fistula area where the needles were to be inserted, or stuck. If I used my doctor-prescribed numbing cream on my fistula to offset the pain from the needle stick, it was washed off at that time.

Chapter 3

The Hemodialysis Session Routine

In this chapter I will talk about what happens once you arrive at the dialysis center and what happens during the hemodialysis treatment session all the way through to the point when the dialysis technician takes you off the dialysis machine. I'll explain some complications that I had and solutions I learned to remedy them.

Before we get started, I want to suggest to anyone who has a very weak heart to please have a detailed and thorough discussion with your nephrologist about whether hemodialysis is the right choice of treatment for you. I say this because nearly everyone I have encountered, who had a reportedly weak heart and was also having hemodialysis treatments in my dialysis center, had very difficult dialysis treatment sessions. Often, their blood pressure dropped so low — after being on the dialysis machine for only 30 minutes — that a nurse would have to stop the hemodialysis treatment and take them off the machine.

On dialysis days, when I first arrive at the dialysis center, I would sit in a waiting room usually just outside of the treatment room. Everyone waited just outside a door until a dialysis technician or nurse called our names and one by one, let us into the dialysis treatment room.

The first thing I would do was step on the scale to take my weight. The scale was set to weigh in kilograms, not pounds (one kilogram = 2.2 pounds). I would write down my weight on the scribble paper provided before giving it to the dialysis technician. Next thing I would always do was wash my hands and my fistula area where the needles were to be inserted, or stuck. If I used my doctor-prescribed numbing cream on my fistula to offset the pain from the needle stick,

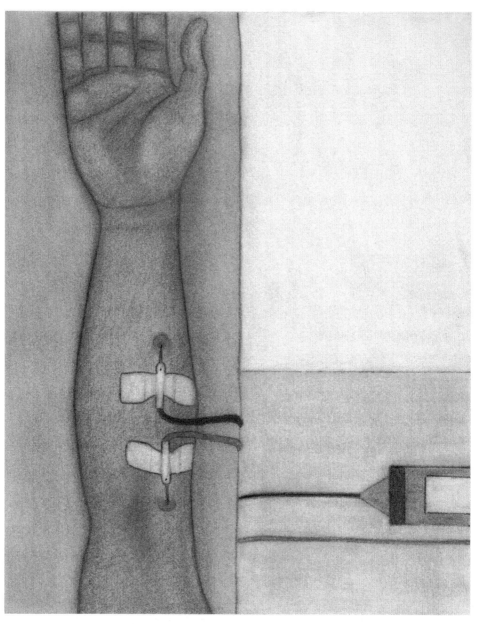

Here is an example of how the dialysis needles are "stuck" once a dialysis patient is ready to start their dialysis session.

it was washed off at that time.

Prior to the technician putting me on the hemodialysis machine, the dialysis technician would always ask the question of the day, "Have there been any changes to your health since the last time you were here?"

Here are some examples of what they wanted to know: Have you had diarrhea? Or a cold? Stubbed your toe? Cut your finger? Are you not eating? Do you have your period? Have you had any medical changes in any way? Your answer may determine how well your dialysis treatment session goes. Depending on my answer, the dialysis nurse would sometimes call my nephrologist. This sometimes resulted in blood samples being taken from my blood line for testing before starting my treatment, or having a change made to my dialysis prescription for that day.

After the question of the day a blood pressure cuff was placed on the arm without the fistula. At this point, the technician would record my blood pressure while standing and sitting prior to sticking my needles.

Once the needle stick was completed, blood flowed through plastic tubing, through the dialyzer, and the treatment began. The dialysis machine is set to take the patient's blood pressure at regular intervals. At the dialysis facility I attended, the machine checked my blood pressure every 30 minutes. They also set an alarm to sound off if my blood pressure went too low or too high, based on the limits my nephrologist ordered.

Once hemodialysis began, the dialysis technician then set the machine to take off the extra fluids I had gained since my last dialysis session. How did the technician know how much extra fluids to take off? This is where my nephrologist's determination of my "dry weight" came in and after a few weeks on hemodialysis I discovered that there was a limit to how much water my body would allow the dialysis machine to remove in one session.

Chapter 4

Dry Weight

In regard to dialysis, a person's dry weight, which is measured in kilograms, is their weight without excess salt and fluid. It was my nephrologist's job to prescribe my dry weight and it's that measurement that the dialysis technician tried to reach at the end of every dialysis treatment.

If your dry weight is 50 kilos and on dialysis day you weigh 53 kilos, the dialysis technician will try to take off three kilograms to bring you back down to your prescribed dry weight of 50 kilograms. This is done by setting the dialysis machine to remove three kilos of salt and water.

My nephrologist would adjust my prescribed dry weight from time to time to compensate for my gaining or losing fat or muscle weight. When I gained or lost fat or muscle, my prescribed dry weight would have to be adjusted to reflect my new, true body weight.

I remember when my dry weight was 65 kilos: I got on the dialysis scale one day and weighed in at 69 kilos. At that time I had already lost the ability to make urine. After my first year on hemodialysis I no longer made urine. According to my nephrologist, continuation of your kidney disease and low blood pressure episodes are the main reasons for losing the ability to make urine. Dialysis then became even more of a challenge since any liquids I put into my body, which included liquids from any foods like fruits or vegetables that naturally contained liquids, could only leave my body by way of vomiting, diarrhea, or dialysis.

That day, I had gained four kilos since my last dialysis treatment. By then, I already knew that I was going to have a problem at the end of my dialysis if I tried to remove all four kilos of excess salt and water.

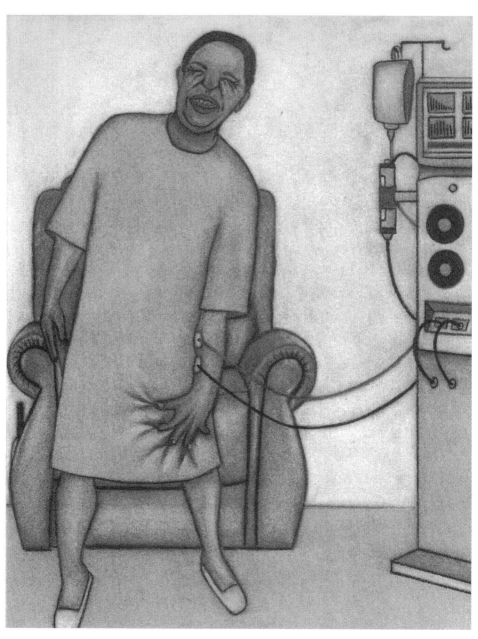

I had a very painful cramp, because my body couldn't handle the machine removing so much salt and water during the prescribed four hours for my dialysis treatment.

I had previously tried to remove four kilos and the results were disastrous. My blood pressure dropped and I had a very painful cramp, because my body couldn't handle the machine removing so much salt and water during the prescribed four hours for my dialysis treatment. The cramp was so painful that I had to stand up from my recliner to put pressure on my right leg to relieve the pain. But that wasn't enough. Most of the pain continued until the dialysis technician came over and injected 200 cc (almost a cup) of saline into my blood line. Saline is sterile, salty water. In other words, the very salt and water they were taking off was now being put back in me in order to correct a low blood pressure episode and muscle cramps, which was being caused by trying to take off water faster than my body would allow within the limited time frame prescribed for my treatment.

At the end of my session the cramp was gone and I left dialysis with my blood cleaned as needed, but not all the water that needed to be taken off could be removed. I learned that my body could only tolerate a rate of three kilos of fluid removed during my prescribed dialysis treatment time of four hours and forty five minutes. Increasing the amount of fluid removal without increasing the time on dialysis meant I would suffer low blood pressure and/or a muscle cramp.

One of the hardest things I did as a hemodialysis patient was controlling how much liquid I put into my body. I could not just indulge in a drinking party where I could lose control of myself because when I returned to dialysis for treatment to remove the extra fluids, I risked having incurred consequences that may be irreversible.

I learned to pay greater attention to the amount of liquid I put in my body and tried harder not to exceed my limit. On days when I'd exceeded my limit, we would only remove what my body safely allowed, requiring me to return the next day to take off the remainder. That meant an extra day on dialysis that week.

Remember, the two important functions of your dialysis treatment are: 1) to clean your blood and 2) to remove excess salt and water. I have seen people come to dialysis with 6-9 kilos of extra salt and water in them. The dialysis treatment would successfully clean their blood but the excess salt and water couldn't be removed safely during their four to five hour dialysis treatment. Very often those people were referred to the hospital. I have seen some of them stay in the hospital for weeks. There were two people I know of who died after repeatedly gaining excess salt and fluid between dialysis sessions. This was called fluid abuse by my nurses.

Chapter 5

The Importance of Monitoring Your Blood Pressure

Let's talk more about low blood pressure episodes and what I learned to do to prevent them from happening during my dialysis treatments. Since I no longer made urine after a year on hemodialysis, my dialysis treatments became more challenging. If I drank more fluids than my body allowed to be removed safely during my prescribed treatment time, but we removed it all anyway, my blood pressure would drop. I discovered how I could help prevent or reverse the occurrence of low blood pressure, especially toward the end of my dialysis treatment.

The dialysis machine is on wheels. I learned to always ask the dialysis technician to turn and face the machine toward me so I could see my blood pressure reading. As the machine removed fluids, my blood pressure slowly decreased. If my blood pressure dropped too low, I experienced severe cramping; dizziness; unconsciousness; fistula clots; and the feeling of being wiped out, or exhaustion. Depending on how low my blood pressure dropped, feeling wiped out could last into the next day.

There was a time when I cramped and/or had low blood pressure for three weeks in a row when I was on dialysis. I thought to myself, "There has to be an easier way."

Taking into account everything I had already learned, I realized that my blood pressure was the key. So I started to watch my blood pressure. I noticed my blood pressure would usually drop the most toward my last hour on dialysis. I already knew that at the end of a good dialysis treatment — after I'd been taken off the machine — my systolic blood pressure (the top number that indicates pressure

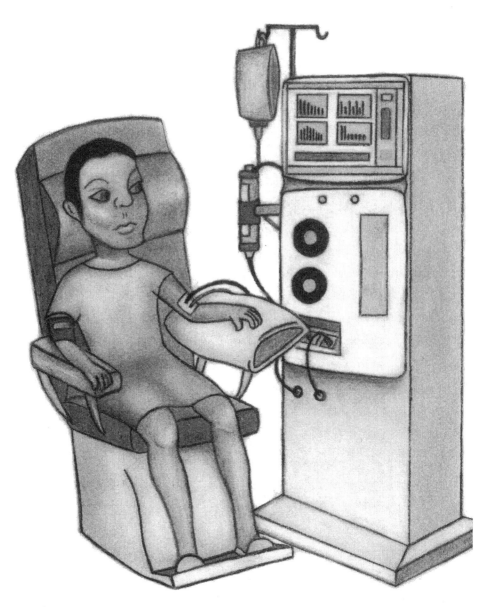

When on dialysis always ask the dialysis technician to turn the machine so you may monitor your blood pressure reading on the display screen.

when the heart beats while pumping blood) usually lands in the range of 110-120. That would be the final blood pressure reading of my dialysis treatment.

One day I noticed that my systolic pressure was at 120 and I had a little more than an hour left on the dialysis machine. So I called over a nurse and explained the situation to her. I told her that if the dialysis machine continued to take off water for the remaining hour that I was going to suffer a low blood pressure episode and/or cramp before the end of my dialysis treatment because my blood pressure was already where my final blood pressure should be.

The nurse completely understood exactly my situation and suggested that she slow the water being pulled out of me. She adjusted the machine but after 15 minutes went by, my systolic pressure had dropped to 110. I called the nurse over again. This time she adjusted the dialysis machine to continue cleaning my blood, but to stop removing water. This worked in my favor. At the end of my session, my blood pressure on that day was 115, right where it needed to be. I continued this monitoring process as needed for my remaining years on dialysis.

Your body may give you a warning that your blood pressure is dropping too low. My warning sign was located at my right pointer finger where I would feel a tiny ache or I would feel the side of my hand suck in. Whenever either one of these signs were present or both were present at the same time I would always get low blood pressure shortly after.

Since everyone's body responds differently, you will likely get a different warning sign like feeling very warm suddenly or yawning, maybe even some of the same symptoms as I had. Once you identify the symptom(s) and they appear, start watching your blood pressure and take action if necessary.

Sometimes I saw that my dry weight needed to be adjusted. When I was eating well and exercising regularly, I gained muscle weight and wouldn't be able to get down to my prescribed dry weight. When I ran into that issue I would ask my nephrologist to adjust my dry weight when he made his rounds at my dialysis center. I would tell him all my woes when he made his rounds.

If I was not eating well or was having diarrhea or vomiting for a period of time, I sometimes lost muscle or fat. During those times my real weight would drop. So when I weighed in at the dialysis center and gave the dialysis technician my weight they noticed this and logged in my weight loss. If the dialysis technician set the machine to my prescribed dry weight without letting my nephrologist know of my weight loss, extra salt and water would be left in my blood. When this happened my final blood pressure would remain high after my dialysis treatment, I would tend to still have some swelling, and I would be unable to drink much without feeling overloaded by fluids.

To get this extra salt and water removed I would have to ask to schedule an extra dialysis session the next day for two hours. After the extra dialysis treatment session, the remainder of the extra salt and water would be removed and my blood pressure would be manageable again.

I used to take my blood pressure medicine with breakfast, lunch and dinner without ever checking my blood pressure. I assumed my pressure was always high and taking my blood pressure medicine on time would control it. I continued this practice until I started dialysis and sometimes found myself dizzy when standing. I spoke to my nephrologist about this and he told me to check if my blood pressure was low whenever I got dizzy and sure enough it was.

Once I started hemodialysis, I made sure I checked my blood pressure before I took my blood pressure medicines. Be very careful when taking blood pressure medicines after a hemodialysis session. A person can pass out if they take blood pressure medicines when their blood pressure is already low after a dialysis session. If my blood pressure was not high, then I wouldn't take any blood pressure medi-

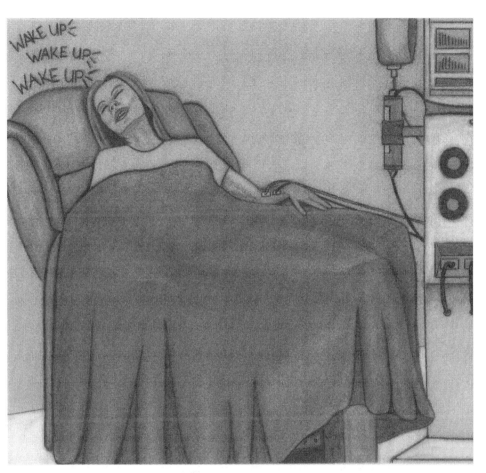

Preventing low blood pressure while on hemodialysis can reduce the risk of low blood flow to the brain, which can cause loss of consciousness.

cine. I have had low blood pressure from my hemodialysis treatment last until noon the following day without needing blood pressure lowering medicines. Be very cautious here.

Chapter 6

Getting Off the Machine

When it was time to get off the machine the dialysis technician would remove one needle at a time. Immediately after the first needle was removed, they would place a cotton gauze ball over the needle's entry point, apply pressure to the gauze and then tape the gauze ball to my arm. They would continue to apply pressure until I could take over applying pressure to the gauze. The same thing happened for the second needle.

I learned to hold and apply pressure for at least 10 minutes before easing up. The main reason I needed to apply pressure and hold for 10 minutes was because the needle created a big hole and a blood thinner was sometimes added to my blood during dialysis. This combination would sometimes make it difficult for my body to form a clot and stop bleeding from the needle stick sites. Once, even after I had applied pressure for 10 minutes, upon removal of the gauze ball, my blood shot out about a couple of feet in small bursts. I panicked the first time it happened and quickly called for my technician.

My technician was sometimes busy taking one of my dialysis neighbors off their machine so help didn't always seem readily available. Everybody seems to come off the dialysis machine one right after another. Eventually, I learned to call for any technician to help me control the bleeding.

A dialysis technician would stop whatever they were doing to come and assist me. They would create another cotton gauze ball for me to apply pressure to the bleeding site. However, they usually didn't stand and wait another 10 minutes with me. They usually resumed their task of taking their other dialysis patients off their machines and I had to wait until they were done and able to assist me again.

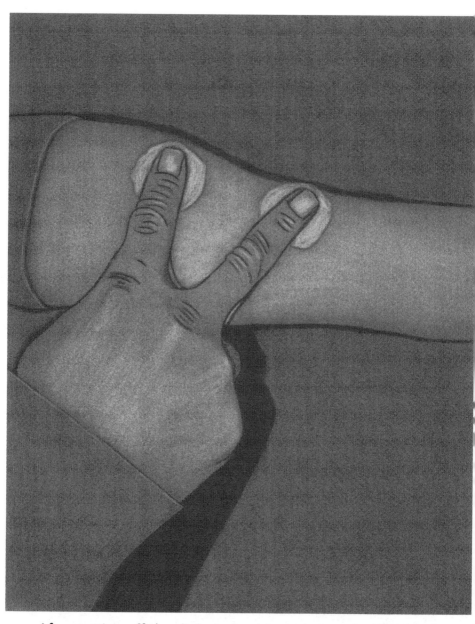

After getting off the dialysis machine, I learned to hold and apply pressure on the gauze balls for at least 10 minutes before easing up.

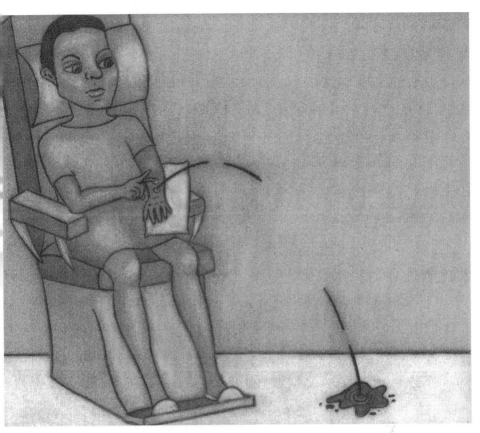

Often while on hemodialysis, you may be put on a blood thinner. When this happens you may find it difficult to create a clot to stop the bleeding once the dialysis needles are removed. When this happens the blood will spurt two to three feet out from you. Nearly everyone on hemodialysis experiences this at some point.

Sometimes it could take 30 to 40 additional minutes. Once my dialysis technician was freed up from taking people off their dialysis machine, they would return to me to make sure I didn't bleed again once I stopped applying pressure. This process was very frustrating. However, it will probably happen to almost everyone on hemodialysis at one time or another.

The last thing the dialysis technician did was take a final blood pressure reading to log in my dialysis record. If my reading was acceptable, I was free to leave the dialysis unit.

I would always leave the cotton gauze balls taped to my skin for at least four hours because if I tampered with it too soon, blood sometimes oozed out, like a slow leak. Whenever this happened I would put a band aid over the point where I was leaking and apply minor pressure for about five minutes. Sometimes I would even put tape over the band aid for a couple of hours.

Chapter 7

Exercise

I think the people who are fortunate enough to survive and start dialysis are blessed. Dialysis is available to artificially extend our lives in the absence of working kidneys. Dialysis, however, is only one piece of the pie when it comes to our overall health and well-being. Diet and exercise are also very important.

A simple exercise like walking has given me many positive benefits. I walked while I was on hemodialysis. At first it was only on non-dialysis days. When preparing for my kidney transplant I increased my walking days to Mondays through Fridays. It really helped me control my blood pressure, sleep better, feel better, and get in shape to bounce back from surgery during the postoperative period.

Today, studies have shown that there are real health benefits to walking for at least 30 minutes a day. These days, I walk for at least one hour, five days a week. This helps keep my blood pressure in the 113/73 range without having to take blood pressure medicines.

Swimming, jumping rope, gardening and almost every activity helps. At one point, when I was still on dialysis and walking five days a week, I told my nephrologist that I no longer felt like I was a dialysis patient. The quality of life benefits of walking helped me feel very similar to the way I feel today with a working kidney transplant.

Chapter 8

Diet

In this chapter I have prepared a fruit, vegetable and beverage schedule to help you.

The schedule will show a variety of fruits and vegetables that are high and low in potassium and phosphorus in case your doctor and/or dietitian have advised you to limit these foods based on your lab results or condition.

The nutritional information in this schedule was prepared by a certified dietitian with the University of Hawaii but I have assembled my own photos to accompany it.

Low- and Medium-Potassium Fruits

Less than 200 mg/serving

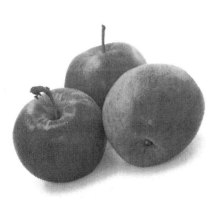

Apple (1 whole)

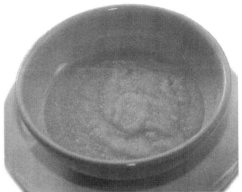

Applesauce (½ cup)

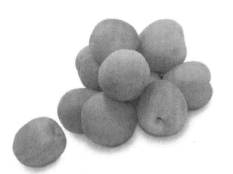

Apricot, canned (3 halves)

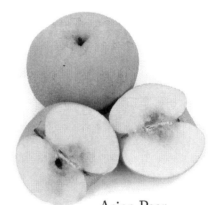

Asian Pear –
Japanese or Korean (1/2 c)

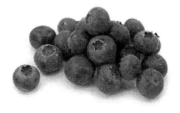

Blueberries (½ cup)

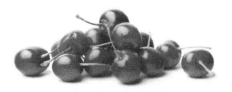

Cherries (10 pc)

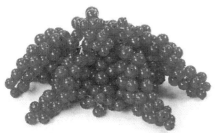

Cranberries (1 cup)

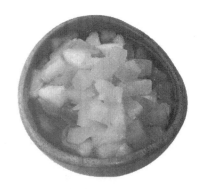

Fruit cocktail (½ cup)

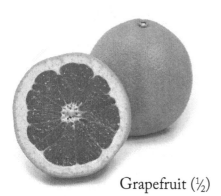

Grapefruit (½)

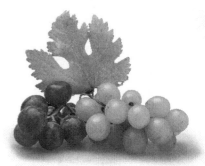

Grapes (10 pc)

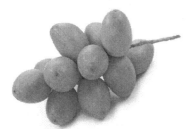

Kumquat, raw (5 whole)

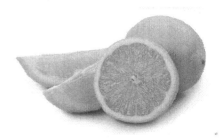

Lemon (1 whole)

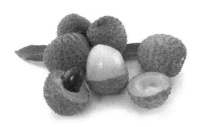

Lychee (10 pc)

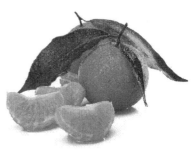

Mandarin orange (½ cup)

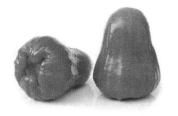

Mountain apple (1 whole)

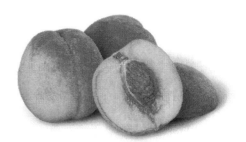

Peach (1 whole)

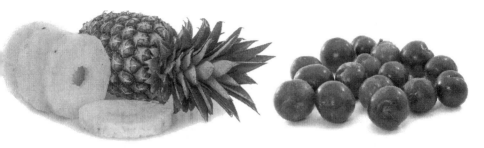

Pineapple (½ cup)

Plum (1 whole)

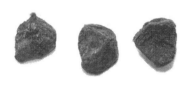

Prunes, canned (5 pc)

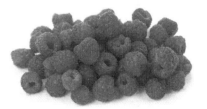

Raspberries (½ cup)

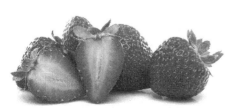

Strawberries (½ cup)

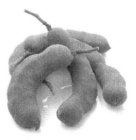

Tamarind (1 fruit, 3"x1")

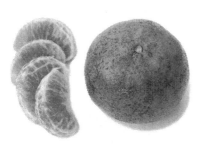 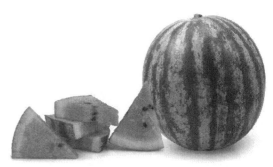

Tangerine (1 whole)   Watermelon (1 cup)

Low- and Medium-Potassium Vegetables

Less than 200 mg/serving

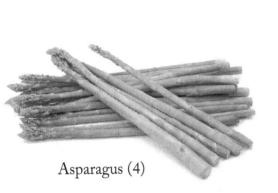

Asparagus (4)

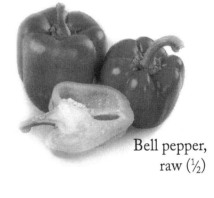

Bamboo shoots
canned (½ can)

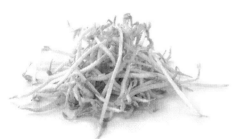

Bean sprouts (½ cup)

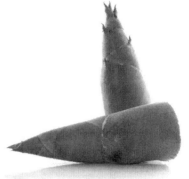

Bell pepper,
raw (½)

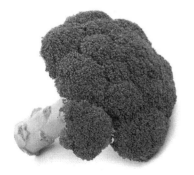

Broccoli, raw (½ cup)

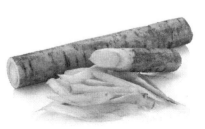

Burdock/Gobo, raw (½ cup)

51

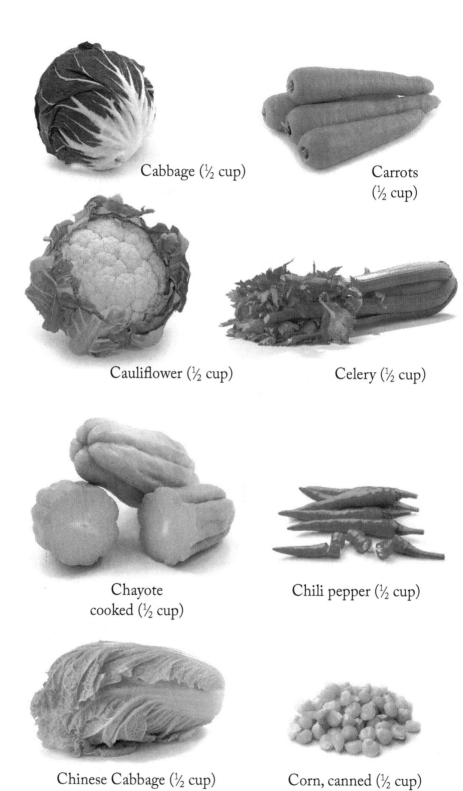

Cabbage (½ cup)

Carrots (½ cup)

Cauliflower (½ cup)

Celery (½ cup)

Chayote cooked (½ cup)

Chili pepper (½ cup)

Chinese Cabbage (½ cup)

Corn, canned (½ cup)

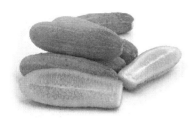

Cucumber (½ cup)

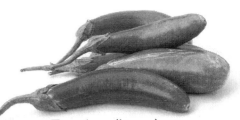

Eggplant (½ cup)

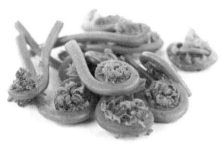

Fern (½ cup, chopped)

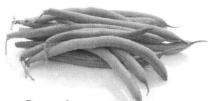

Green beans (½ cup)

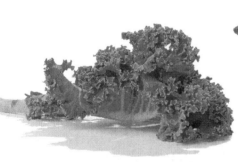

Kale (½ cup)

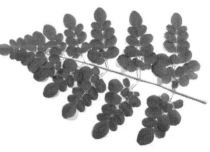

Marungay leaves (½ cup)

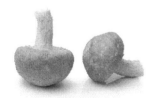

Mushrooms (button or shiitake), raw (½ cup)

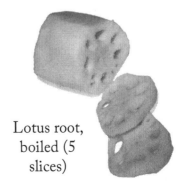

Lotus root, boiled (5 slices)

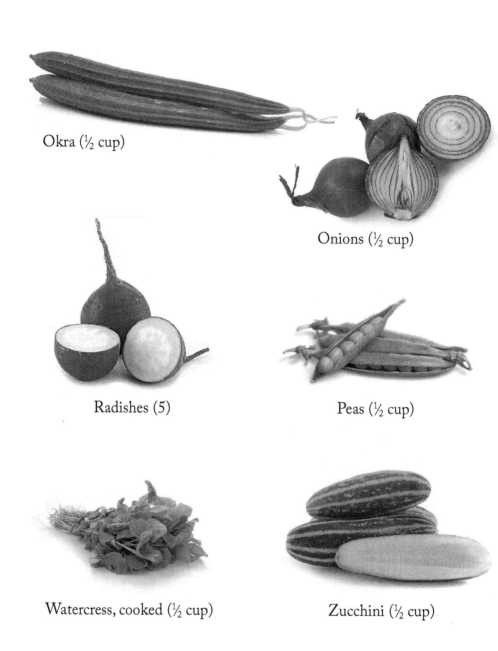

Okra (½ cup)

Onions (½ cup)

Radishes (5)

Peas (½ cup)

Watercress, cooked (½ cup)

Zucchini (½ cup)

High Potassium Fruits — Limit or Avoid

Less than 200 mg/serving

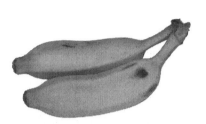

Apple Banana (1 whole)

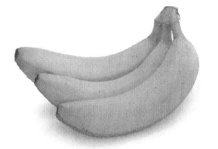

Banana (½)

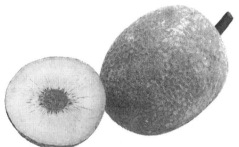

Breadfruit (¼)

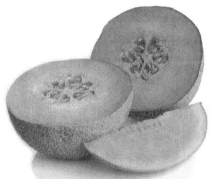

Cantaloupe (½ cup)

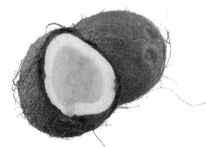

Coconut, raw (¼ cup)
Coconut milk (½ cup)
Coconut water (½ cup)

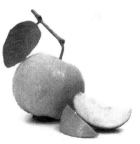

Guava, raw (1 whole)

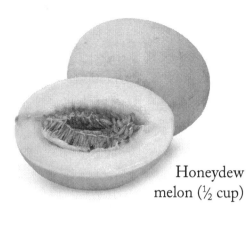

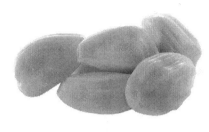

Honeydew melon (½ cup)

Jackfruit (½ cup, sliced)

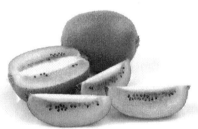

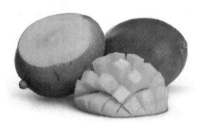

Kiwi (1 whole)

Mango (½ medium)

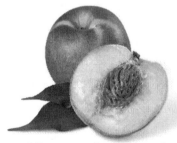

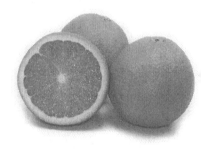

Nectarine (1 medium)

Orange (1 medium)

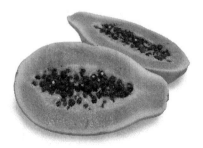

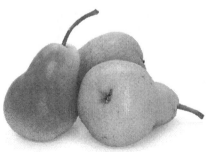

Papaya (½ small)

Pear (1 medium)

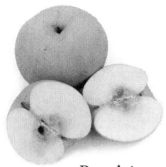

Pear, Asian
(1 whole, 3 ⅜"x3")

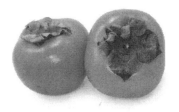

Persimmon, raw
(1 whole)

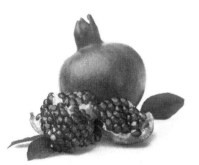

Pomegranate, raw
(1 whole)

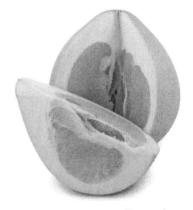

Pomelo, raw (½ cup)

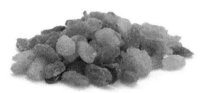

Raisins, snack box
(1½ oz.)

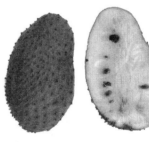

Soursop (½ cup)

High-Potassium Vegetables — Limit or Avoid

Less than 200 mg/serving

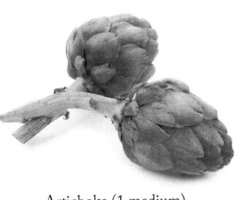

Artichoke (1 medium)

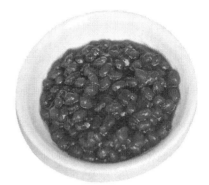

Azuki beans (½ cup)

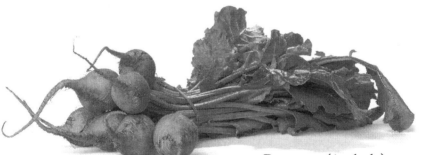

Beet, raw (1 whole)

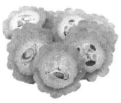

Bitter melon (½ cup)

Brussels sprouts (½ cup)

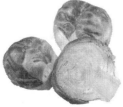

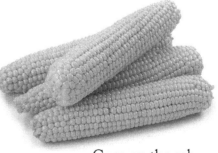

Corn on the cob (½ cup)

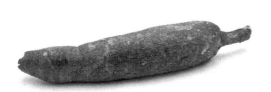

Cassava (½)

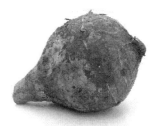

Dasheen (½ cup)

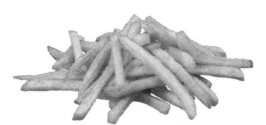

French fries (½ cup)

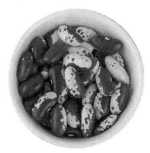

Kidney beans (½ cup)

Lima beans
(½ cup)

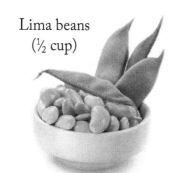

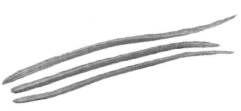

Marungay pods (½ cup)

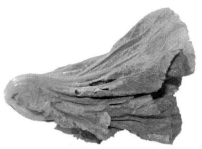

Mung beans (½ cup)

Mustard cabbage (½ cup)

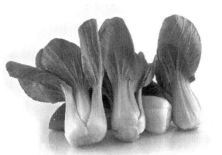

Pak (Bok) Choy (½ cup)

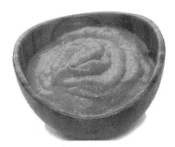

Poi (½ cup)

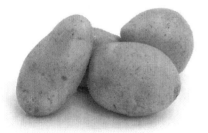

Potato, boiled (½)

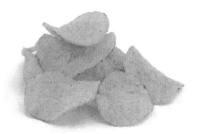

Potato Chips (15 chips)

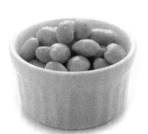

Soy beans(¼ cup)

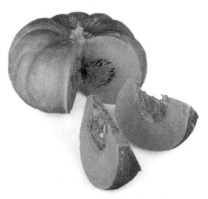

Squash, Acorn (¼ cup)

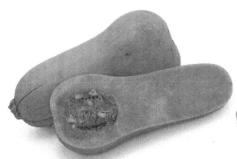

Squash, Butternut (½ cup)

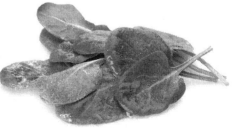

Spinach, raw (1 cup, chopped)

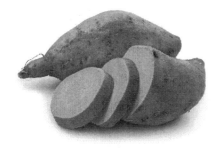

Sweet Potato (½ cup)

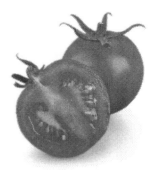

Tomato (1 medium)

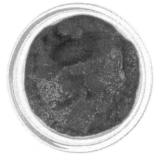

Tomato paste (2 tbsp.)

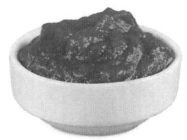

Tomato sauce (½ cup)

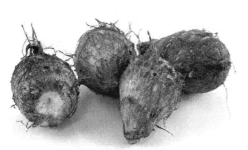

Taro (½ cup)

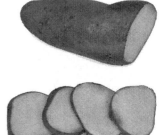

Yams (½ cup)

Low- and Medium-Potassium Drinks

Less than 200 mg/serving

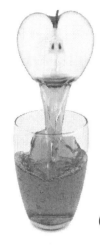

Apple
juice
(½ cup)

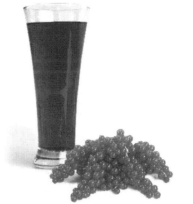

Cranberry juice (½ cup)

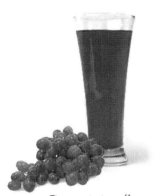

Grape juice (½ cup)

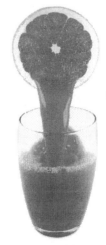

Grapefruit
juice
(½ cup)

Guava juice
(½ cup)

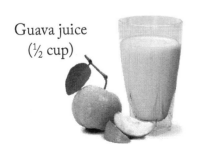

Lilikoi/Passion
Fruit juice
(½ cup)

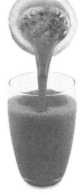

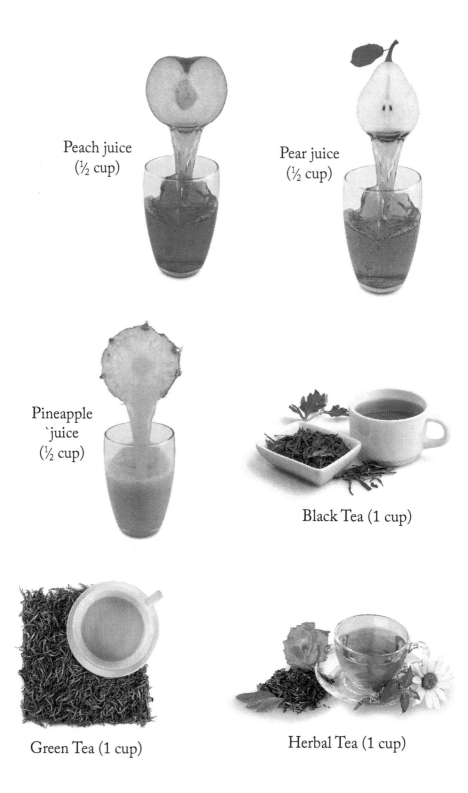

Peach juice
(½ cup)

Pear juice
(½ cup)

Pineapple
`juice
(½ cup)

Black Tea (1 cup)

Green Tea (1 cup)

Herbal Tea (1 cup)

Limit or Avoid

High in Potassium and/or Phosphorus

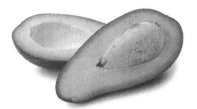

Avocado, Hawaiian variety

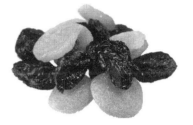

Dried Fruit

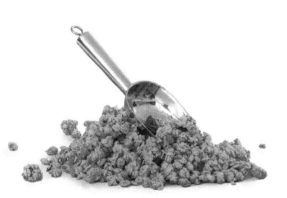

Granola

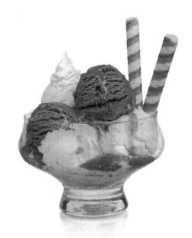

Ice Cream

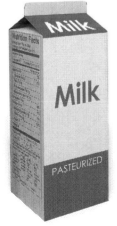

Milk

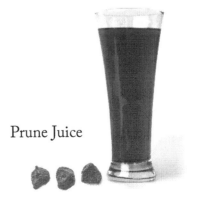

Prune Juice

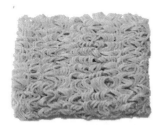

Saimin

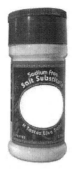

Salt Substitute

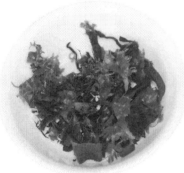

Seaweed

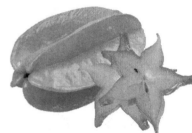

Star Fruit
(very toxic to kidneys)

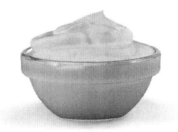

Yogurt

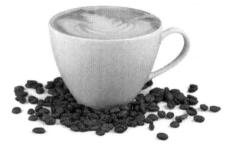

Latte or Cappuccino

Foods High in Phosphorus

Some of these foods may be added into your diet in small amounts.
Check with your Registered Dietitian Nutritionist.

DAIRY

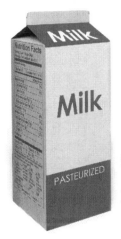

Milk

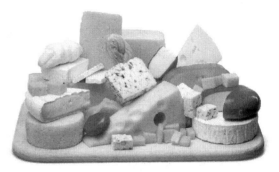

Cheese

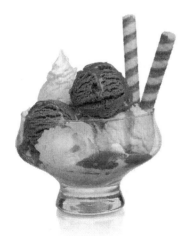

Ice Cream

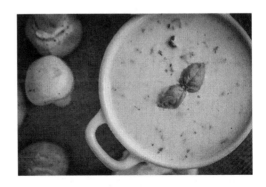

Cream Soups

Foods High in Phosphorus (cont'd)

Some of these foods may be added into your diet in small amounts.
Check with your Registered Dietitian Nutritionist.

BEANS, NUTS, SEEDS

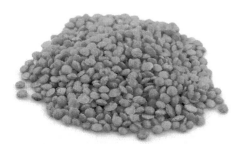

Dried Peas and Lentils

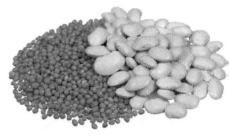

Canned and Dried Beans
(e.g. kidney, azuki, mung)

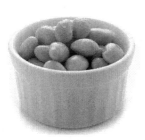

Edamame (soybeans)

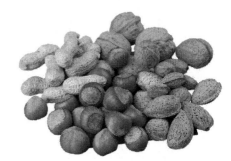

Nuts and Seeds

Foods High in Phosphorus (cont'd)

Some of these foods may be added into your diet in small amounts.
Check with your Registered Dietitian Nutritionist.

GRAINS

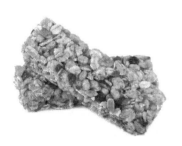

Granola and Breakfast Bars

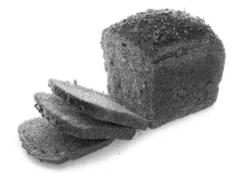

Whole-grain Breads

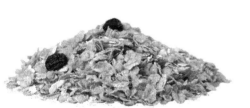

Bran Cereal

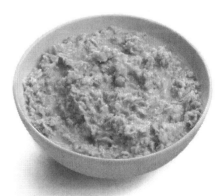

Oatmeal

Foods High in Phosphorus (cont'd)

Some of these foods may be added into your diet in small amounts.
Check with your Registered Dietitian Nutritionist.

OTHER

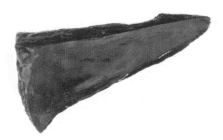

Organ Meats
(Liver, kidney)

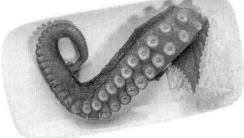

Tako (Octopus)

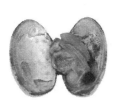

Clams or Oysters

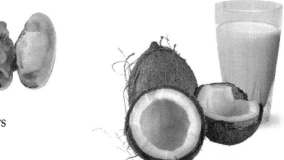

Coconut Milk

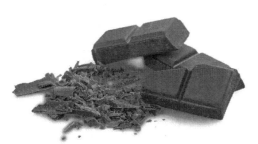

Chocolate

Foods with Added Phosphorus — Avoid These Foods

Phosphorus is added to many processed foods. Added phosphorus is absorbed by our bodies more than phosphorus that is naturally found in foods like whole grains, fruits, vegetables, and dairy products.

Look for words that begin with "Phos" to help you identify added phosphorus in ingredient lists on foods (e.g. Dicalcium **phos**phate, potassium tripoly**phos**phate).

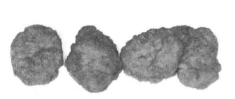

Chicken Nuggets

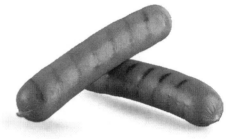

Hot dogs, Cold cuts

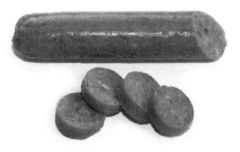

Sausages (Vienna, Portuguese)

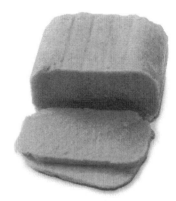

Canned Meats

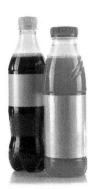

Some bottled and canned iced teas, coffees, colas

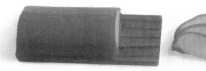

Fish cake and Imitation Crabmeat

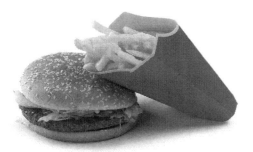

Many fast foods

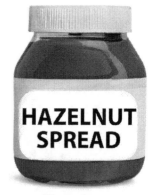

Chocolate —
hazelnut spreads

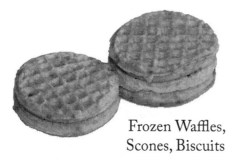

Frozen Waffles,
Scones, Biscuits

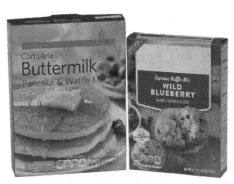

Cake doughnuts

Boxed mixes (pancakes, muffin,
cornbread, etc.)

Made in the USA
Columbia, SC
12 October 2020